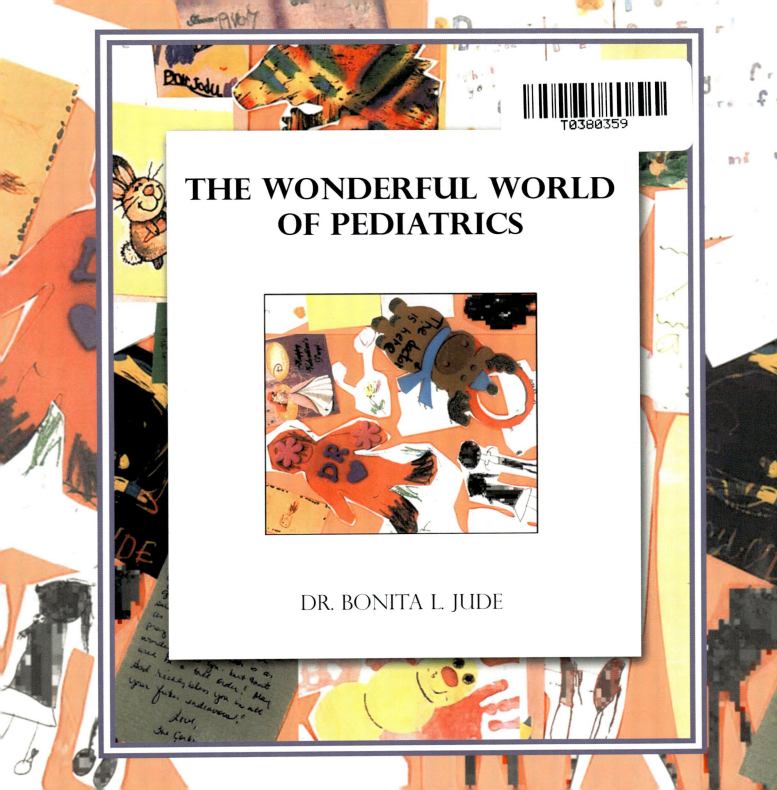

# THE WONDERFUL WORLD OF PEDIATRICS

DR. BONITA L. JUDE

To order additional copies of this book, contact:
Xlibris
844-714-8691
www.Xlibris.com
Orders@Xlibris.com

ISBN:   Softcover        978-1-6698-5119-6
        EBook            978-1-6698-5120-2

Library of Congress Control Number:     2022920975

Print information available on the last page

Rev. date: 02/01/2023

# THE WONDERFUL WORLD OF PEDIATRICS

## *Out Of The Mouth Of My Many Angels*

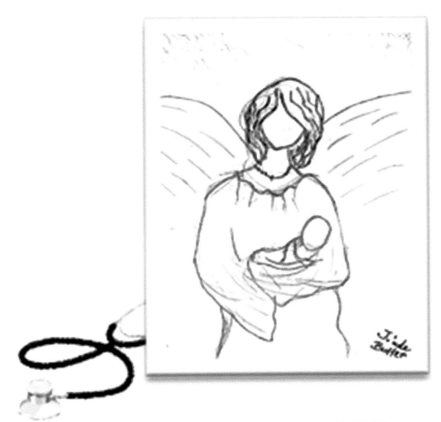

## DR. BONITA L. JUDE

Layout and Design by Tammy Marshall

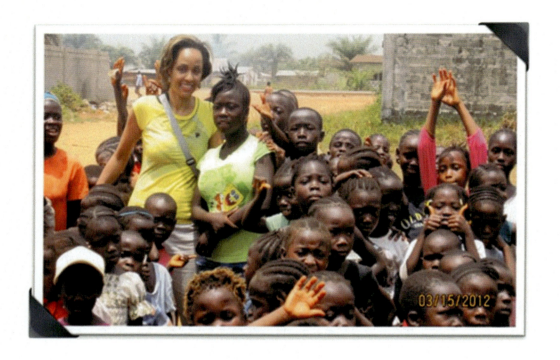

Then people brought little children to Jesus for him to place his hands on them and pray for them. But the disciples rebuked them. Jesus said, "Let the little children come to me, and do not hinder them, for the kingdom of heaven belongs to such as these.

Matthew 19:13-14

# DEDICATION

I dedicate this book to two very important people in my life who helped made my medical journey a reality.

My Grandmother, Jeannette Louise Howard Cooper-King, was the first Black Nurse to receive the highest award in nursing, the Florence Nightingale Award. She was a true trailblazer, paving the way for others like myself to enter the medical profession. My Grannie, as I affectionately called her, was my inspiration to go into medicine. She demonstrated to me (effortlessly) there is nothing more significant in life than to help alleviate suffering for our fellowman and to be the hands and feet of our Lord and Savior, Jesus. I have been trying all my career to reach up to her achievements, but I still have a long way to go. I am so thankful to my Grannie for raising me to be the Christian medical provider that I am. I love and miss you dearly.

Dean Stephen Risen, Dean of Student affairs, Hahnemann School of Medicine. Without Dean Risen constant encouragement, counselling, and tutelage I don't think I would have made it out of medical school in one piece. He took a particular interest in my success. I am forever grateful to him. I apologize because I think I cause his hair to turn gray by the time I graduated from medical school. He cared and was always there; to encourage me through the failures and rejoice with me through the successes. It was only fitting that I requested him to robe me as I walked across the stage at graduation. Thank you for being my guardian angel during a very challenging period in my life. But it is worth every strand of gray and more because I am living my "purpose".

All of this is futile without the Lord Jesus Christ being my Savior. Thank you for the ultimate sacrifice... The Blood.

# TABLE OF CONTENTS

Introduction                                    7

The Road Less Traveled                          9

Residency 1993                                  11

Mission Accomplished                            15

Out of the Mouth of Angels                      16

Acknowledgement                                 70

About the Author                                72

# INTRODUCTION

Aww, to be like a child again. The innocence, the imagination, the hope and dreams, the discoveries, the limitlessness, the cut, bruises, teacups and dress up are all so priceless.

I have always had an affinity for kids, even when I was a child. I often took care of my baby cousins and fell in love with them.

Babies are so innocent, they smile often (except for certain circumstances, like diaper changes or need to be fed). Mostly, they are always so happy to see me, and stare at me as if listening to every word I speak. I started experimenting with kids, like taking care of their ouches, when I was still in elementary school. I would emulate what I saw my grandmother do to treat wounds and cuts. I love seeing her squeeze the pus out of an abscess- the more pungent, the better. I realize I have now lost a few readers, but one either loves this line of work or not; there is a special gene for this stuff (just joking). My tail always wagged when left in charge of my baby cousins. I would not only play "doctor" with them (they were my first actual patients) but also line them up and play school. I eventually played matchmaker and decided to marry two cousins off by the time they turned four.

Being around children, I feel free to be myself without making any pretends. I never feel judged, and we have a fantastic time, fill with laughter and awe. Our imagination is never limited because there are no boundaries around endless possibilities. More importantly than anything, when I am around kids, I feel the tangible presence of a loving Heavenly Father, who is unconditional love. And then when I look into a newborn's face shortly after birth, I can sense a soft glow radiating all around them. I often tell the new parents that their babies just left heaven sooner than we did.

The field of Pediatrics was my calling from the beginning, even when I was in my mother's womb. Though it was the most difficult accomplishment of my life, and numerous times I doubted it, I knew it was either Pediatrics or nothing.

I have now been in the field for over two and a half decades, and I do not regret that decision. Especially when told I did not have what it takes to become a doctor or when colleagues would challenge every decision I made simply because they only saw my skin color and not my medical decisions. I was predestined for this field, so I kept my eyes on the One who fashioned me for this profession. I also knew every day I would work in the pediatric clinic would be a big "recess" break in clinic. It has not always been fun, especially when an innocent child's life ended. Even in that sad moment, I learned an indelible lesson to improve the world for the next patient.

My patients have been branded on my heart for life, and they have touched me in one way or another. I will always be grateful I got to participate in the lives of these little ones who do get to inherit the kingdom of heaven just by being.

I hope you enjoy a few quotes I have collected over the years from my patients, the true stars.

## THE ROAD LESS TRAVELED

Residency was a big blur, mainly because as a resident, we were so sleep-deprived that it did not allow for everyday life. Being on and off "call" for years on end, with a 2-week break between the years, only allowed one to breathe, eat and keep working. But I relish those years (okay, maybe not when I had not slept for over 36 plus hours and still had to be able to make life or death decisions) because I was finally working in a profession I have dreamt, prayed, and cried over for almost all my life.

There were many patients I came across over the years but a few, who I still think about almost every day and whose "Barney" watch I still carry. I have never been so challenged mentally and spiritually after being so close-up front to death, as I experienced during Residency. At times I questioned if I was even making a difference in just one child's life. Seeing a 3-month-old baby die in the PICU due to a congenital brain malformation or a 5-year-old girl succumb to B-cell acute myeloid leukemia made me question my choice. I believed I wanted to be challenged so I went into Residency thinking I wanted to be a Pediatric Intensivist, but I knew after a year of residency I could not see another child die without a part of me passing along with them. To be able to help a broader range of children for a career span, I knew being a General Pediatrician was the right fit for my longevity and sanity. I do not regret a moment of that decision.

As I stated in the beginning of this introduction, the field of Pediatrics was my calling. A loving heavenly Father puts giftings, talents and desires in every seed at the time of conception. When we are born, prayerfully we are birthed in an environment which can nurture, nourish, support, and encourage these God-given purposes.

I am so grateful I was born in such a family, a natural family and a family of educators, friends, and a community.

Another deep passion of my is medical missions to developing nations. I see the extreme effects of an environment that does not foster healthy living or lack of provisions for children. Being a pediatrician allows me to help a larger population of children born in this situation for no fault of their own or even their family. Sometimes I feel I am putting a bandage on a gapping chasm, but then I convince myself at least that is a bandage that the child did not have at that moment. So being a General Pediatrician serves a greater good than just my desire.

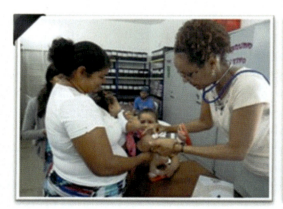 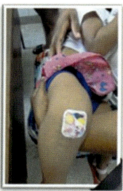

*Putting a bandage on a child in an impoverished area of Brazil.*

## RESIDENCY 1993

The reason I wrote this book was to focus on the patients, the true gift of God. So enough of me, and now I present these darling angels.

I must expand on the one patient I alluded to, who give me my first "Barney" watch. For those who do not know who Barney is, Barney is or was a purple dinosaur who rocked the 80s and 90s (RIP Barney).

I walked into the PICU (Pediatric Intensive Care Unit) to start rounds that morning and there she was, hooked up to over ten tubes going in and out of her body. Harmony was a 3-year-old who unfortunately was born with a congenital heart malformation. Her heart did not develop properly. I was the Intern assigned to her. We did not hit it off right away. Recovering from cardiac surgery can be frightful. I knew she was in pain, was scared, felt alone and far away from home. Harmony was being cared for by her aging grandparents.

When Harmony transferred from the PICU to the regular Pediatric unit, we were best of friends. I remembered arriving a bit early every morning before rounds started so I could be the first to wake her up. I remembered a few times she would be up with her eyes peeking through the hospital bed railing, saying softly, "Dr. Doo, Dr. Doo" as she could not say Dr. Jude. Harmony and I were inseparable between my other responsibilities and patients care. I would take her to the hospital cafeteria (when allowed) and walks around the hospital. Unfortunately, Harmony had a relapse and had to go back into the PICU. I spend the night with her, though it was not my night on-call. She had now occupied a part of my "mommy's heart' that no one else had. Thank God Harmony recovered, and after a few months, she regained her strength and was healthy enough to get discharge from the hospital and move back to Hawaii, where she and her grandparents lived.

Every medical resident knows the first two years of residency are the most challenging, atrocious, brutal period of one's life. The professional, emotional, and mental challenge can sometimes be over whelming. Because of my strong faith in the One who called me from conception, I knew I would succeed. But at times I needed Harmony to keep me afloat as much as she needed me to check her laboratory values, volume input, output, blood culture, etc. Now it was time to say goodbye for maybe forever as I did not know what would happen to this now 4-year-old who was leaving to cross the Pacific Ocean for a distant island I might never visit. It was around the Christmas holiday, and I volunteered to take her and her grandparents to the airport, mainly because I wanted to spend as much time as I could with Harmony. Her family were not the wealthiest people and did not have a lot to offer. Still, at the airport, her grandparents blessed me with a monetary gift that Harmony's Cardiologist told me later was monumental and a big sacrifice knowing their family financial situation. They said in the card, they wanted me to go back home (to Maryland) and be with my family for the holidays because I had told them I could not afford to go home on a resident salary. I held Harmony so close to me before letting her get on the plane until I felt her heartbeat perfectly in harmony with mine.

I kept in touch with Harmony over the years, as her grandparents periodically send me pictures, so I could see her grow up into this beautiful middle schooler.

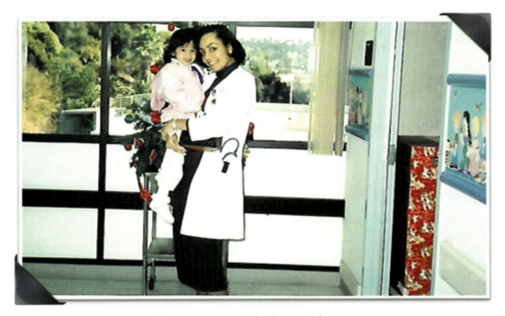

*Harmony and I during residency*

Nine years later, in 2002 after that tearful day at Los Angeles International airport I jumped at the opportunity to attend a medical conference in Honolulu, Hawaii. I contacted Harmony's grandparents and we set a date and place for our reunion; it was determined to be near the beach overlooking Diamond Head. On the appointed day, as the car approached me waiting on the beautiful shores of Waikiki beach, Harmony leaped out of the car without hesitation and jumped straight into my arms. My baby was all grown up. She still was her spunky, happy self, enjoying every second of life. Due to her heart defect, she was smaller than an average 12- year-old, but still had a personality larger than life. I placed a heart-shaped necklace around her neck, as she had also brought me a bracelet, earrings, and charm in the shape of the national Hawaiian flower - the Hibiscus.

Here she was, my forever diamond, overlooking Diamond Head, sparkling brighter than ever, smelling with the sweet fragrance of the Hibiscus flower.

Two years after our reunion in Honolulu, I received the dreaded phone call from Grandma informing me that my Harmony was now 100 percent healed with a perfect heart jumping all over the grounds of heaven, radiating brighter than ever. Hallelujah.

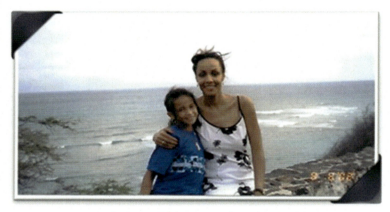

*Harmony and me in Hawaii, our last earthly encounter*

"He will wipe away every tear from their eyes.
There will be no more death, or mourning or crying or pain,
for the old order of things had passed away."

Revelation 21:4

## MISSION ACCOMPLISHED

The year was 1998, I had just finished Residency and was working at my first paid job as a pediatrician. It was exciting that finally, I would be working in a profession I had cried over, sweated over, even bled a few times over, endured all my life to begin, and now that day was finally here. And so, it begins.

Not sure when I knew to start capturing these quotes from my patients, but I am so glad I decided one day to buy a Composition copybook. I carried that book around for two and a half decade and would write down these treasures. I hope it makes you laugh and ponder the unadulterated gems that comes out of the mouths of babes.

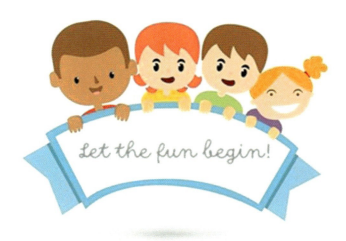

# OUT OF THE MOUTH OF ANGELS

Dr. Jude, the 1<sup>st</sup> patient is waiting in the dinosaur room.

**Advise from a 3-year-old, if you want to get a boyfriend.**

Naomi was a 3-year-old who came to see me because her mother was concerned about the color of her stool. It was green. I examined her and after an extensive history I realized Naomi was an unusual toddler because she loved vegetables. The color of the stool was due to her excellent intake of vegetables. I commended her for her dietary intake and reassured her mother that all was well.

Naomi was also a precocious toddler. While finishing my notes, she tells me she is three years old and has a boyfriend. I tell Naomi I am 30- something years old and do not have a boyfriend. She tells me that I need to eat my vegetables and then I will get a boyfriend.

*I am thinking to myself; Naomi probably loves watching Veggie tales and she thinks Larry is a heart throb, but a 30-year-old needs more than a cucumber for a life mate.*

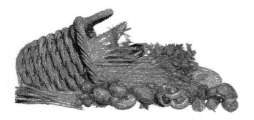

**A Future Pastor**

Every child is always terrified of coming to the Doctor. They first want to know "am I getting shots." I am so grateful at my clinic; as pediatricians, we DO NOT have to give the kids shots.

I always reassured the kids, 'I am the good person, I do not give shots" (sorry nurses, you all get stuck with the worse job, making these innocent babies cry. So, I make sure to give my nurses a good Christmas gift). The parents usually feel sorry for the nurses, so they try and shift the blame back to me by making me feel guilty for ordering the shots. Well, I quickly shift it back to the parents and tell them "You all brought the kids in here," light heartedly.

Rachel is four years old and needs her booster shots to start Kindergarten when she turns 5. As I finish the visit and was about to leave the room for the nurse to come in to give her the vaccines, she told me "May the peace of the Lord be with you."

*I did not know what to do next, do I bow down and start confessing my sins to this little 4-year-old, and ask her for forgiveness since I was responsible for inflicting pain on her innocent gentle soul, or do I have her anoint my head before I leave the room.*

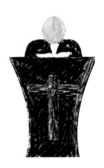

## Future Pediatrician

Four-year-old Hannah always loved coming in to see me. Her mother told me Hannah would put on her mother's heels, placed her toy stethoscope around her neck, and pretend to be Dr. Jude.

*That warmed my heart because I never realized what a physical impact I was making on these little angels. As stated earlier, the road traveled in getting this degree was exceedingly arduous, so when I am at work, my main concern is making the correct diagnosis and treatment and making sure I treat my family with respect and love. I did not realize my fashion style was also just as crucial to my 4-year- old female patients.*

Another fan was 3-year-old Emma. Emma's mother told me that Emma had named her Barbie doll after Dr. Jude because "she was so nice and sweet." Mom went on to say to me that I should be honored because Emma does not name her dolls after <u>anyone</u>.

*I love my job.*

Another note of importance, this was in 1998, before the turn of the century when female made up less than 30% of doctors in the USA and even less percent being a black Doctors (less than 3%). So having my white patients pretending to be me, shows we genuinely live in a great country, where Dr. Martin Luther King statement is active; "we are judged by the content of our character and not the color of our skin."

If I am ever having a bad day or just heard terrible news on the TV, or the dog peeped on the carpet or having a bad hair day, just being with my patients turns the entire atmosphere around for good. Just ask this next patient.

**Lover Boy**

Five-year-old Nathan told me during a visit for a bug bite, he always kisses the Christmas tree every year. When I asked why he did that, he says he did it because it is the "Kiss-mas" tree.

*I am sure his parents are so proud of their son.*

**Future 'Ladies' Man**

Jean came in for her annual physical examination, accompanied by her mother and two-year-old brother, David. While I was examining Jean, I felt a pair of hands rubbing my legs. I looked down and there was David, "I like your stockings Dr. Jude" he said. The mother profusely apologized and told me she does not have the time to wear stockings because she is at home taking care of a five and two-year-old, so David was not use to the look or feel of stockings.

*I have never blushed so much, especially not due to a 3-foot-tall male.*

**Brain Washed Kids**

I was counselling seven years-old Matthew and his 5-year-old brother on the harmful effects of watching excessive TV has on the developing brain. His mother charms in and stated she only lets them watch Public TV because it does not have commercials. She felt commercials brain wash people.

Matthews then ask, "how can you wash the brain and which soap would you use?"

*I will let his science teacher explain the composition of brainwash soap.*

I have had the honor to serve this wonderful country by working in military medicine over the last two and a half decades. I have such high respect for the men and women who wear the uniform and put their lives on the line so I can enjoy the freedom to live out my dream by working in a profession I adore.

The rest of the patients are taken from these Heroes' dependents/ children. So, enjoy as I salute our future.

**A Lost Security**

Five-year-old Jason came in because he was sad. His mother stated he had just gotten rid of his security blanket ten days ago. Jason corrected his mother and stated it was only three days ago, "now I only have the rest of my life to go without security."

*Jason might need to talk to Dr Phil to plan his life trajectory.*

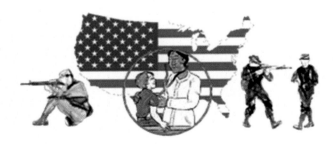

### 3-year-old Tommy

I asked him what does he like? He stated, "I like the Hohoho man."

*Get it? Santa says Hohoho.*

### Future Stephen King Producer

Six-year-old twins accompanied their 3-year-old sister for her annual well visit. The 3-year-old had developed allergies. The mother explained that she was raised with cats and had never developed allergies as an adult, so she felt her kids would be okay if she got them a cat or a dog. One of the twin's eyes grew big when his mother said that. He stated, "I did not know you were raised by cats; didn't you have a Mommy and Daddy?"

### Future Kentucky Fry Chicken Owner

Eleven-year-old-Nathan came in for his sport physical. I always get a dietary history to assess how healthy it is. I asked Nathan what he likes to eat. He states, "chitlins and fried okra.".

*I was speechless after that answer because I had never gotten that response before. I think Nathan family is from down South and loves good ole southern cooking.*

Five-year-old Adam was asked during his annual physical examination if he ever talk to strangers. Adam looked me straight in the eyes and said, "No, because if you do, they can trick you and make kid stew."

*That convince me to become a vegan.*

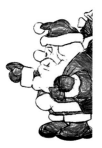

**Future Albert Einstein**

Four-year-old Alex came into the clinic for a questionable bug bite on his arm. I examined the bite marks on his skin and told him it was probably an insect bite. I asked him if he saw a spider in his room, which could be the culprit. He looked at me and told me, "A spider is not an insect, it has 8 legs."

*Please don't take my medical degree from me Dr. Alex.*


**Our Future is in GREAT Hands**

Five-year-old Michael came in for his annual physical. After reviewing his immunization record, I informed him he did not need any shots. Pastor Michael replied, "I already knew that because I just prayed !!"

Five-year-old Arron. When asked what he would do if you got lost, within seconds, he responded, "call God."

The world is getting evil everyday so I must make sure my patients are prepared to face the danger.

Fifteen-year-old Daya was asked during her physical examination what she would do if a stranger approached her and asked for help finding a lost dog who just ran away. She replied, "I would smile and say no thank you and leave." After her exam I called her 9-year-old brother from the waiting room to also be examined. I asked the same question, and believe it or not, he said the same answer, as the mother smile with such deserved pride.

*I can retire now, knowing that the world is in good hands.*

I was running late during the clinic that day, about 20 minutes so I profusely apologized when I entered the room. 5-year-old Matthew was waiting to be seen and stated, "This is okay Dr. Jude, I have to sit an hour in church, so it's all good."

The future is in good hands with 8-year-olds like Sarah. She came in for an annual physical. Concentrating on oral hygiene, I asked her if she brushed every day. "Yes, I do brush, floss every day, then I read my Bible."

*You go girl!*

Five-year-old Malaika was asked during her physical examination if she watches TV. She stated that she used to watch Lion Guard (the new Lion King) but doesn't anymore because Honey Dagger said a bad word. With great trepidation I asked what he said. Malaika said, "he said **duh** !!!".

*I can now retire peacefully and pass on the baton to this younger generation. There is great hope.*

**The Next James Bond**

Seven-year-old Reggie dislocated his right thumb, was seen at an Urgent Care and had his thumb placed in a splint. He came in to see me for a follow up visit. I was not impressed with the splint he had on, so I told him I must use a splint that is more adorable. Macho Reggie asked me, "does it have to be adorable?"

**Sassy sister**

Five-year-old Ashley came in for a physical, accompanied by her mother and 3-year-old sister. I asked Ashley what she would do if she went to the store and got lost. Ashley answered: "yell for help." Sassy 3-year-old sister charms in and said: "and then find yourself."

Another sassy sister. 4-year-old Tanner came to the clinic with his mother and 2-year-old sister. After greeting the family, I asked the mother what was bothering Tanner today. Out of the corner of the room came a sneaky voice from his 2-year-old sister; "His penis hurts."

**The Beauty of Innocence**

His father brought 5-year-old Christopher in for a school physical in preparation for kindergarten. Part of the visit is going through anticipatory guideline. I must ensure these precious babies are ready to face this big, bad world.

Question: *Do you wear a helmet when you ride your bike?*
Christopher's answer: yes.
Question: *What do you do before you cross the street?*
Answer: Look both ways.
Question: *Do you ever talk to strangers?*
Christopher hesitated before answering and looked so stunned, before he said: *No, I don't even know one.*

Eight-year-old Anastasia came in for her school physical. I asked her what she would do if she went to the store with her mother and got lost. She replied, "I would go to a nice lady and ask for help. Do you want to know how I know she is nice?" she asked. I was sitting at the edge of my seat now with bated breath. Her answered, "because she is really old."

*FYI kids- strangers danger, regardless of age or personality assessment.*

## Kids and Medications

Eight-year-old Kelsey developed an ear infection that needed treatment with antibiotics. That antibiotic needed to be taken with food for better absorption. I instructed the mother and Kelsey to take the medication with food. Kelsey looked confused so I asked her if she had a question. She replied: "every time I eat, do I have to take the medicine?"

*Maybe Kelsey will be a future Spokesperson for Weight Watchers.*

Seven-year-old Owen came in for evaluation for allergies symptoms. I diagnosed him with Allergic rhinitis and prescribed Zyrtec. He did not like the taste of the liquid medication, so I told him I could prescribe tablets. I assured him he was a big boy and could swallow a tiny pill. "Zyrtec is a very small pill, about the size of my pen tip", I told him (as I showed him my pen). Owen then asked me, "why do you have a pill on your pen."

Ten-year-old Perry came in for an infected left big toe. I prescribed antibiotic and told him he had to take the medicine for seven days. Perry then asked me what the side effects were from this antibiotic. I have never been asked this question before by a patient, not a 10-year-old, so it took me by surprise. I asked him I did not understand his question. Perry replied, "I mean, will I get twitching of the eyes, nails turning blue, teeth falling out?"

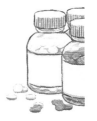

Yes, I love being a pediatrician, but... **I am not a fan of teenagers** (not sure who is). **I believe my favorite age group** is the 4- and 5-year-olds. They can communicate effectively; they are cute as a button and think they have the world figured out. Unlike the teenagers who think they have the world figured out, only to realize they are WRONG and barely keep up with hygiene.

A 17-year-old came in for an asthma evaluation. In the room next door was a newborn crying. I asked the teenager how he felt being in the same clinic with Dinosaurs stickers on the wall and babies crying all over. He replied: "old." I felt good about myself because I finally got him to talk. It might have been one word, but he uttered an audible sound at least. I was on a roll, so I dared to ask another question, but I felt we had connected, so I asked him: "well, how do you think I feel." Yes, I opened that proverbial can, and being true to his age he replied: "like dirt."

*Did I mention I do not like teenagers; not all, just most. Some are angels, from another planet. I ordered a few more shots for Mr. 17-year-old that day.*

**Introducing the Next Cover Model for GQ Magazine**

A 14-year-old male came into the clinic for episodes of wheezing and coughing. Though it was summertime, he had on a few layers of clothing. For me to auscultate his lungs, I had to go under those layers. While trying to pull the 2nd layer of his bulky T-shirt up, he started screaming: "You're giving me a wedgie."

*Oops, sorry. His mother reprimanded him for wearing so many layers in the hot weather.*

## Mr. Philosopher

Four-year-old Adam was asked during his physical exam if he ever talk to strangers. His response, with a lot of confidence, was: "I only talk to the strangers I know."

*I just had to hug him after that response.*

The following family had just deployed from Hawaii, so 4-year-old (my favorite age group) Michael came in for his annual physical. I went over his diet history and asked him what he likes to eat. Michael informed me he loves fruits, especially pineapple; he drinks milk and water and loves pineapple meat.

*I been to Hawaii once, but I do not recall being offered pineapple meat. But then maybe Jared (the next quote below) from Jurassic Park and Michael discovered a new species of meat that roamed the earth before time.*

## The Founder of Jurassic Park

Four-year-old Jared told me during one of his visits that he was a dinosaur expert. He started naming all the different types of dinosaurs, names even I could not pronounce, but this 4-year-old had no problems going through the list. Jared told me about Stegosaurus, so I asked if they were in the Jurassic Park movie. He informed me that Stegosaurus were here before Jesus was born, and Tyrannosaurus had small arms because Jesus's Father made them like that.

*I had to look up what Tyrannosaurus was. For us adults with limited brain cells, unlike the 4-year-old with an IQ of 200, that is a T. Rex.*

Five-year-old Dawn told me when she went to the Zoo last week, she saw Dinosaurs and Elephants.

### Transient Environment in Military Medicine

Military families are constantly being deployed. It can be a bit emotional because once I have gotten attached to the families and vice versa, it is time for the families to move to their next duty station.

Five-year-old Kent had a wart on his big toe and came in for treatment. He asked me if warts come from Lizard pee. I told him to call Jared from Jurassic Park for the answer. I treated his wart and instructed his mother to bring him back in six months for a follow-up. Kent stated his dad needs to go to Iraq for six months, so when he returns from Iraq, that would be a reminder to come in to see me.

*Bless his soul for caring for this burden in his little 5-year-old mind.*

### The Comfort of Growing up in a Military Home

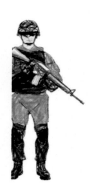

Five-year-old Justin came in for the annual visit. Going over anticipatory guidelines and questions, I asked, "what would you do if you got lost." Justin's answer: "ask someone." "Someone like who?" I asked. Justin: replies, "someone who is nice." How do you know if someone is nice? The answer, "a human." I started laughing hard, then came the solution of all answers; Justin said; "I got it, A MARINE."

*Oorah*

Please read this article that was published in the military newspaper "Stripe" in April 2011. Certain patients, like Harmony are not just patients but more like family. I fell in love with John Jr when he first entered the examination room. He was so polite, precocious, and cute. His mother would always correct him when I asked him a question; he was only allowed to answer with a Yes, Ma'am or No, Ma'am. I LOVE southern hospitality. Like southern sweet tea, the world would be a lot nicer and sweeter. I also received a plethora of artwork from John Jr with each clinic visit.

Enjoy this article; hopefully, the readers can appreciate the sacrifice our military families give to our great country year in and year out.

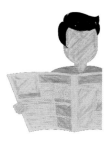

# The Goodbye List and Dr. Jude
## Special farewell eases move for military child

By Ingrid Murray
Special to the Stripe

My son is sitting at the kitchen table working on our moving calendar. We will be PCSing from Fort Belvoir, Va., to Redstone Arsenal, Ala. He draws two rows of seven blocks and writes the dates in. As he is writing he says, "Mama, I am 5 and we will be moving again and I will have lived four places. I am only 5 and that's a lot of moves." Yes, I say to myself, it is a lot of moves.

John Jr., then says, "There. I am done making the move to Alabama calendar. Now I have to make my goodbye list."

I wipe my hands on a dishtowel and walk over to the table. John Jr., explains to me that he is writing down the names of people he loves at Fort Belvoir and he is going to say goodbye to. Then when he sees the person he hugs them, they sign the list and he will take a picture of them for his Fort Belvoir memory book.

He gets a clean sheet of paper and then tells me I can't look at his goodbye list until he is finished. I go back to the kitchen. I hear him sounding out names and see him erasing and then writing again.

As I put supper in the oven, I hear him proudly proclaim, "Mama, I am finished...you can come and see my goodbye list." I walk over and he shows me the list and I smile. I see many names I expect: his "best friend forever and ever" Chance Heck, his friends at school and church, his Fort Belvoir AWANA teacher, Ms. Rosie, the school and post librarian, and then a name I didn't expect to see — Dr. Jude, his pediatrician. I ask about her name and John Jr., tells me in that matter-of-fact way of 5-year-olds, "Dr. Jude loves me. I love her and when I get sick, she gets me better, even when I throwed up really, really bad. Do you remember that time, Mama? Dr. Jude makes me take shots sometimes I don't like, but I still really love her. When you love someone and you are going away, you have to tell them 'goodbye.'"

John Jr., then puts his list next to the calendar and ask me to help mark the days he will begin to say goodbye. Each day we writes a persons name. Then we have one name left — Dr. Jude. John Jr., looks at me and asks, "When can I tell Dr. Jude goodbye?" I explain that Dr. Jude is very busy with sick children and since he is healthy, we may not be able to see her. John Jr., then tells me matter of factly, to write her a note and let her know he is going away and wants to tell her goodbye and, "then she will see me."

The days go by and we begin to mark off our list and take pictures and get lots of hugs. John Jr., takes the goodbye list everywhere and it has become rather ragged. Each morning he makes sure to put it in his backpack, and then after school he unfolds and studies it. We have one week left, he comes home from school and as he is working on his homework, says to me, "So Mom, I still need to see Dr. Jude for my goodbye list." I again explain that I don't think we will be able to

# Saying goodbye

From Page 2

them a hug and then say goodbye."

So we head up to the clinic and wait to see Dr. Jude on her supper break.

Dr. Jude then walks in the room.

John Jr's., face lights up as does Dr. Jude's, and they are in there own world. Dr. Jude asking questions and John Jr. replying excitedly about Alabama and the rocket ships.

Tears begin to fill my eyes. I have to bite my lip to stop the tears from falling.

I hear John Jr., telling Dr. Jude about the goodbye list and he knew that she would want to see him and hug him and say goodbye. He tells her that I said she would be too busy with sick kids but that he "knew that you love me and would miss me if I didn't tell you where I was going." She agrees and thanks him for meeting with her. They continue to chatter about any and everything.

I then begin to wonder if this one goodbye would even matter five or 10 years from now.

As memories of Fort Belvoir fade and new ones are created, would this one goodbye to Dr. Jude matter? Goodbyes are hard, but ask any Army spouse, they are much harder when you have a child. Your heart aches for them.

The Army has so many programs to help families and children with PCS moves, but sometimes I learned it is the people, like Dr. Jude, who makes the biggest difference — the people who are committed to serving the military families and especially the children.

In that instant I realized it, that five or 10 years from now wasn't important — it was the here and now. Dr. Jude knew that. Here was a 5-year-old military child who was moving again. It was going to be hard — new friends, new school, new home, new stores and even a new pediatrician. She could not change any of that, but she could take time, her own supper break, to help him with his goodbye list and maybe, just maybe, make the goodbye a little less sad.

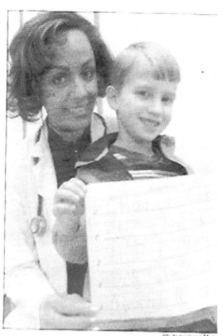

Photo by Ingrid Mills

**Dr. Bonita Jude of the pediatrics clinic a DeWitt Army Community Hospital at For Belvoir, Va., takes time to sign to the good bye list of John Jr., as he and his family pre pare to PCS to Redstone Arsenal, Ala.**

Dr. Jude then took out her pen to sign her name by where John Jr. had printed her name. He then gave her a big hug and a sticker and I took a picture. I then to get a hug and as we left the office, John Jr., was skipping down the hallway of DeWitt Army Community Hospital clutching his goodbye list with a big smile on his face.

Thank you United States Army for having great people like Dr. Jude, DeWitt Army Community Hospital, serving the military families.

*Thank you, Ingrid and John Jr. Miss, and love you all.*

The things I have learned from the patients over the years are more than I learned in medical school and Residency combined.

Nine-year-old Alyssa informed me that eating asparagus would turn my urine green. I was not about to correct an innocent, cute 9-year-old. I would if she was a teenager.

**Spelling Bee Winner**

Studies have shown if kids are read to from the beginning (even before birth), they develop better verbal and reading skills, have higher IQ and their families are more intact.

Four-year-old Alisa. I asked her to spell her name. Her response: A-L-I, with a dot, S-A.

Five-year-old Liam injured his right foot playing around at home. He came in to see me. I informed the Mother I would order an X-ray to rule out a fracture. Liam kept asking what an X-ray was. I explained that it is like getting a picture of your foot, but Liam still looked confused. Then he said: "I know Dr. Jude; it is like when Curious George broke his bone and had to go to the doctor."

*Twelve years of post-graduate studies could not have explained getting a radiograph as precisely as 5 -year-old Liam.*

## Mix Drinks in Pediatrics

Six-year-old Nathaniel came in for a physical. After getting his diet history, I asked him what does he drink? Nathaniel response: "I drink Gatorade, which is like water but with dust."

Eight-year-old Sharon came to the clinic with her father for a headache. I performed a Neurology exam, including check the function of the Olfactory nerve (which determines the ability to differentiate smells). I usually have the patient close their eyes and allow them to smell different items. Because there is an abundance of alcohol pads, I had Sharon smell the pad. Her father almost melted in the seat after her answer. "It smells like something Dad drinks."

We use a communication device in the clinic called Vocera. It allows me to call the nurses and order immunizations, medications, etc.

A family of 2 kids, 2 and 4.5 years old, came in for vaccines, so I used the Vocera to call the nurse to prepare the vaccines. The 4.5-year said "cool" and looked amazed at the functionality of this device. So, I tried to explain to them that it works like a Walkie-talkie from the 70s. They still looked puzzled, so the mother attempted to explain what a Walkie-Talkie was. She said: "you get two empty cans, like a peach can and a green bean can, put a hole in the middle and run a string in the middle of the cans, and then you can talk with your friends at a distance." The 4.5-year-old bells out, "no, no, let's use beer cans."

Seven-year-old Austin was asked what he likes to drink. He answered, "I like all drinks except beer."

Four-year-old Rowan was asked during his preschool physical what he likes to drink. "COCKTAILS," Rowan said. I turned to the mother with a look of total shock, and the poor mother looked like she wanted to hide under the chair, while she quickly explained, "it's cranberry juice, fruits, and seltzer."

*Okay.*

## The Beauty of Sibling Rivalry

Eight-year-old Jason came in for treatment of a cyst on his right upper eyelid. When I asked what happened to his eye, his 5-year-old sister stated he scratched his eye. Jason immediately replied: "no I did not; go with me, it's my eye."

Four-year-old Jane was asked during her physical. Do you have a dog? "No." Do you have a cat? "No, I have a sister."

I was seeing 3-year-old Coletta for her annual physical and the mother wanted to know what to do to stop her from sucking her thumb. I informed the mother that the bitter stuff does not work. Coletta's 5-year-old brother immediately shouts, "hot sauce will work."

Five-year-old Ashley tells me, "My brother is a peanut, and I love peanuts."

**Result of the New Math Being Taught in the 21st Century**

8 Eight-year-old Adam, a 3rd grader came in for refill on ADHD medication. I asked Adam what today's date was to assess his memory function. His response: "Zero dash 4 dash 11 dash 16."

*I asked in human language what that means: April 11, 2016.*

Five-year-old Albert came in for his Pre-Kindergarten physical. I asked him, how high can you count to? Albert answered: "Zero."

I asked another 5-year-old the same question. I called this patient Kareem Abdul Jabbar (the answer is found in his name). Kareem was sitting down when he started counting. 1,2,3- while moving his hands up. Then he stood up: 4,5,6,7. Then he stood on the chair: 8,9,10, 11,12. "That's as high as I can go Dr. Jude."

*I asked for his autograph after that because when he makes it to the NBA, I had evidence; it all started in the Doctor's office.*

The following patient statement is dedicated to my sister who was a Middle School Math teacher for 33 years in the Public School system. Enjoy this one Sisie.

Eleven-year-old Albert came in with his mother for an evaluation for a rash. The rash was a quick diagnosis, so I started talking to the mother. She tells me she has four sons, and her father has four girls. I informed the mother that the father determines the gender of the child. I briefly explained the role of X and Y chromosomes and the inheritance from Mom or Dad. The mother was so intrigued that she turned to her son to find out if he had learned about the

Xs and Ys chromosomes. Albert replied, "yes I have I've made it to coordinate planes."

*I'm thinking to myself, did I skipped that lesson in Middle school, I called by sister that night and she informed me it was teaching from the "new" math. Good, I can keep my degree.*

### Presenting the True Stars - The Parents

There is a fact in Medical School that Pre-Med students avoid going into Pediatrics because they do not want to deal with the Parents. I love my parents; they make me laugh just as hard as the kids. Pre-Med students love the kids but do not like the Mama Bear personalities. I tell the residents, and new doctors always listen to the parents. They are with their children 24/7. They know their kids. If a mother tells me she feels something is wrong, I try and go the extra mile to find out that "something," despite normal findings. There are a few Munchausen or overly zealous parents, but most know their children and have acceptable concerns. Here are a few examples.

Now for the Mom's joke or acknowledgements. Moms can do no wrong. After examining Bradley's ears, I informed the mother that her child's ears were clean. She replied: "good, because I am not a Q-tip Mom."

*Can someone from Earth please explain what a Q-tip is. Is her hair made of cotton?*

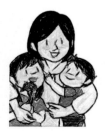

Twelve-year-old Xavier came in for this annual physical. I asked him if he plays any sports. He stated he wanted to play football. His mother immediately stated (to her son) "the reason you cannot play football is that you have poor posture. If you work on your back posture, then you can play football."

*I wonder if Walter Payton or Joe Montana 's mothers give them this same advice.*

Five-year-old Aiden was brought into the clinic for complaints of headache. His mother informed me that she has migraines, and so does her mother. Aiden looked so puzzled and asked his mother with wide eyes, "wait, you have a mom?"

Nine-year-old Clinton came in for 'flu-like' symptoms. I told the mother his symptoms were consistent with a viral upper respiratory infection, so he did not need an antibiotic. He would benefit from fluids, rest, and fever medication- as required. The mother charms in and states, "yes, and also R & R." Clinton replied, "rest and relaxation." Mom stated, "no, rest and read, if you have to be out of school, no electronic, you will rest and read."

*I wish we had more parents like this Mother; the world would be so orderly. And the parents say "AMEN."*

Seventeen-year-old Barbara came in for her annual physical. Her weight was a bit elevated. I instructed her she needed to exercise more. She tells me, "I am so out of shape, even the asthmatics pass me on the track using their inhalers." She goes on to share she wants a private trainer like how her grandmother has. The mother informs her daughter, "your grandmother has one because she is a Silver sneaker, and it is free with Medicare, are YOU a silver sneaker?"

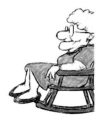

*I guess Mom told her.*

Fourteen-month-old Baby Chang is brought in by his mother, who has a lot of questions. She asked why her baby sweats especially on the scalp at night. I instructed her to decrease the layers of clothing and blankets at night. She then asks why the baby sweat is not salty. I asked her how she knew it was not salty. She stated the baby's grandmother wipes her hands on his scalp and then tastes it.

*Does anyone out there want to take on this question. I was so shocked, it left me speechless.*

Nine-year-old Joan was asked during her physical what she likes to drink. Joan answers, "kids' wine." Her mother immediately explains it is Cranberry juice and Ginger Ale. After which I hung up the phone from Child Protective Services.

Eight-year-old Katie was asked during her physical if she would ever go to the swimming pool by herself. She answered no, but her 6-year-old brother shouted, "she gets to go places by herself." Her mother immediately tried to correct the situation by stating, "she goes to the mailbox by herself, which is right in front of the house."

Nine-year-old Maya came in because she was experiencing foot pain. I diagnosed her with flat feet and notice she was wearing Converse sneakers. I told her she needs shoes that have more arch support and then asked if she always wore these shoes. Maya replies "I just wear whatever Mom gives me."

*I had to get Mom from under the bus.*

Fifteen-year-old Becky came in for allergy symptoms. I explained to her I was going to prescribe a nasal spray, Flonase, which will help with the nasal congestion. Becky immediately asked, "what is a nose spray." Her mother answered, "a spray you put in your nose."

*Way to go Mom, I could not have explained it any better.*

## Mama Bear Meets the Pastor

Four-year-old Mary came in on Monday with a cough, right after her birthday party, which was held two days earlier. Her mother said a child came to the birthday party sick with Croup. She informed me that the child's mother was a nurse, "figure that", angrily, Mom said. Mary said, "but at least he said Happy Birthday nicely."

Seven-year-old Christopher was asked during his annual physical what chores does he must do at home. Chris answers, "I know how to burp on purpose." His mother immediately states," he does do chores, he gets fined if he burps on purpose, and if he does extra-work, he will get paid."

*I gave her a 'high five' as they left the clinic. The world would be much better, safer, less polluted with Moms like this. Love you, Moms.*

A Hispanic mother brought in her 2-year-old son, Xavier, concerned that he does not talk. Mom stated she speaks English to him at home, but he spends a lot of time at his aunt's home, who has a dog. I asked if she speaks Spanish to Xavier. The Mom asked "who, the dog?"

**The Love of a Kid**

Four-year-old Brice was asked during his annual physical if he knew how to write the alphabet.
Brice: "Yes, I can write also write Brice; B-R-I-C-E." Brice replied, "I can also write "Mommy loves Brice."
I was so impressed that a 4-year-old could write a complete sentence, so I asked him to write it.
Brice wrote: M-O-M ♥ B-R-I-C-E

I also love when the Dads bring in the kids. When I walk into the room and see only the Dad with the kid, I know that appointment is going to be a short visit. The Dads usually have no questions, they do not know how many poop and peep diapers there are, do not know how many ounces of formula the baby drinks in a day, they usually feel the kids, especially the boys are over exaggerating their symptoms. They want to check the box, make sure they have asked all of Mama Bears questions, and leave, so they can get back to protecting our country and killing the bad guys. (Sorry if it sounds sexist, it is not, just my experience over the years, knowing there are always exceptions where the roles are reversed).

I also try and make the dads feel comfortable, especially when I observe from their uniform; they are part of the Marines/Special Forces/Navy Seal/Ninja forces. Here they are, looking so uncomfortable, physically fit in their uniform, walking in carrying a 5-pound diaper bag.

These visits are not all about poops and burps. I am an avid sport fan, so I talk to the dads about sports, like who will make it to the Super bowl, how many rings does Tom Brady has, what affect Kevin Durant Achilles tear has on his future, will the Nationals get another run at the World Series. In the end, the diaper bag is forgotten on the chair, so I typically must run down the hall to catch up with the dads before leaving the building.

Twelve-month-old Ruth was brought in by her father for a cough. The Dad stated he treated the cough with Desitin.

*Lesson #1: Desitin is a cream used to treat diaper rash.*
*Lesson #2: If it was Dimetapp that was used, over-the-counter cough medications are not approved for this age group.*
*Lesson #3: In a world where Dads are absent or missing, I applaud these fathers for taking an active role in their children's lives. I encourage Dads to keep bringing their kids in. I promise that we will laugh together and learn together.*

Four-year-old Tyra was brought in by her father for cough and fever for 1 week. Apparently, the father was also sick and stated he had been sick as a dog. Immediately Tyra stated, "you are not a dog, you are a Daddy."

Five-year-old Kailey came in for a diffuse rash. She was very talkative and precocious. I told the father he had a cute talkative daughter. He stated "yes, she is just like me'. The daughter charms in "it is not just you, it is God."

Five-year-old Robin was noted to be at the 99th percentile on her growth curve. The Dad stated she was going to play basketball and that he played forward. Robin asked, "so how would someone play backward?"

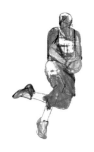

Eight-year-old Joshua is brought in by his parents for questionable pneumonia. The Mother informs me of Joshua's Past Medical History, to include a Heart murmur, Epilepsy and… The father abruptly interrupts and said, "no he does not have Epilepsy." The mother reiterated, "yes, he does have epilepsy." The father said, "you mean my son reads backwards?" We all laughed, as the mother said; "Epilepsy not DYSLEXIA."

*I LOVE the dads. Okay, I'll lay off the dad jokes, for now.*

Okay, one more Dad joke.

Thirteen months-old Hunter was brought in by his father because Hunter was having an asthma exacerbation. I treated him with a nebulizer treatment, which helped, but he continued to wheeze. I told the father I needed to give him a dose of oral steroids, but it was one of the worst- tasting medicines. The father chimes in to say, "Don't worry about that. Hunter will tolerate the steroid because he eats his poop."

*Barf, barf, barf, or maybe I need to call Child Protective Services.*

A bonus one for Dad.

Her father brings in 7-year-old Jackie for her annual physical. Going over safety questions, I ask Jackie if she talks to strangers. She stated she had never met one. I asked her father if there were any guns in the house. He replies, "there are none in the house." Jackie replies, "yes, but we have knives."

**Dr. Google has a Competition from Nickelodeon**

I asked 7-year-old Charlotte about her diet history during her wellness visit. I learned she does not drink milk and does not eat any dairy products. I educated her that her bones need calcium to stay strong and healthy; if she did not have enough calcium, she could develop Osteoporosis when she gets older. She immediately screamed out, "o no." So, I asked her if she knew what Osteoporosis is. She replied, "no." I explained to her osteoporosis causes bending over of bones and fractures. She shouts back to me that she did learn about Osteoporosis in the Nickelodeon magazine.

*I could have kicked myself for spending all that time and money getting a medical degree when all I had to do was grab a few editions of Nickelodeon magazine.*

**Some Kids are so Precocious, it is Scary**

Three years-old Jessica came in for a well-baby visit. I should not call it a well-baby visit because Ms. Jessica could carry on a conversation with me, so I asked Jessica rather than ask the parent for the answers. I asked her what she likes to eat. As she reached for a handful of M&Ms, she said, "I do not like junk food."

*Does anyone want to hire her to sit on the FDA Board of Nutrition?*

Four-year-old Winter came in with a pacifier in her mouth. I tried to convince her that pacifiers were only for babies and not 4-year-old big girls. She informed me that she has tried to get rid of it, but the pacifier keeps saying, "come and get me."

Five-year-old Adam came in for his annual examination. I asked what his future ambitions were. He answered, "If I was President, I would have people listen to God's rule."

I asked 6-Year-old Luis what he does before he crosses the street. Answer- I look at "North, South, East and West."

**Then Others are so Honest**

Nine-year-old Scarlet came in for her annual physical and a vision screen. I took her to the Eye chart (Snellen) and told her to cover one eye and read the line I was pointing to. Scarlet quietly asked me, "can I keep my other eye open?"

Four-year-old Susy. I asked her what she would do if she went to the store with her parents and got lost. She answered, "I would cry."

Eight-year-old Henry, I asked him what he would do if he went to Toy-R- Us with his mother then suddenly, he could not find her. Henry replied, "I would kind of panic and then I would look around."

Five-year-old Deborah came in for a physical. Going over safety questions, I asked her if she would ever go to the pool by herself. "No, I don't know how to drive". I then asked if she sat in her car seat in the back of the car. "No, I don't sit in the trunk, I sit in the seat behind Mommy's seat."

I asked 6-year-old Nancy what was on her Christmas list. She answered, "I cannot write."

During 10-year-old Mark appointment, I asked if he brushes his teeth daily. He answered, "I do it more than I don't do it."

*At least they are not teenagers.*

Five-year-old Mary was asked if she is having any problems sleeping. She said, "yes, in the morning, my nose is stuffy, so I pick it out."

*I made sure to wear gloves before examining Mary.*

Jacob came in for his 5 -year-old well visit. I told his mother Jacob might be the tallest of her sons. On the growth chart, Jacob was at the 95th percentile. I asked the mother if she could recall where her older son was on his height percentile. Mom replied, "I don't know where he is". Jacob immediately replied, "he's in school."

*I love the honesty of kids. This quality is one of the top reasons I chose to work with kids for life.*

## My Fan Base

*I love my patients; I see them like my babies. Hopefully, the feeling is mutual, but not all the time.*

Six-year-old Alex accompanied his 8 months old sister for her well baby visit. While examining little Rhea, Alex kept coming to the examination table to see what I was doing. His mother kept redirecting him to sit on the chair and to give me some space to properly exam Rhea (this happened in 2007, before the 6-foot pandemic guideline). After the final time of redirecting Alex, Mom said; "I know you love Dr. Jude and want to be near her, but you have to give her some space." Alex immediately replied; "I don't love her that much to want to marry her."

*My proverbial balloon popped!!*

I do not know if this next patient is a fan, but I am concerned about his future escapades.

Three-year-old Zachary came in because his mother was concerned about the trajectory of his urine stream. My advice to the mothers is, please ask their husbands about this problem before bringing in their sons. The dads usually have the correct answer way before I do. After examining Adam genitalia, I hear Adam tell his mother that he likes the doctor touching his penis because she has cold hands.

*I have no comments or picture to go along with this capture.*

Eight-year-old Allison came in complaining of left foot pain. After examining her, I realized she had sprained her left ankle. I wrapped her ankle with an ace wrap and explained that Allison needed to limit physical activities for the rest of the year (it was only a few days before the school's Christmas break). She kept smiling and appeared happy with my service. She whispered in her mother's ear, "can I give her a penny?"

*I guess I can retire now.*

Four-year-old and 17 months old sisters came in for their wellness visits. I completed the 4-year-old physical first, then called for the 17 months. Their mother placed her on the exam table, so I walked over to start the examination and said: "hello little pumpkin." The 4-year-old yells, "Her name is NOT PUMPKIN, it is Chanelle." I immediately answer, "well she's my pumpkin," followed by dead silence. Then I heard the 4-year-old ask in a guilty voice, "can I be your pumpkin also?"

**Another Cute Fan, Who Cannot Keep Her Hands Off Me**

Ten months old Courtney was brought to the clinic for a complaint of cough for a few days. I felt a wet finger up my nostril within seconds of hearing clear air flowing through her lungs. I usually close my eyes when listening for heart and lungs sounds; it allows for better clarity and less distractions (until the finger intrusion).

*I LOVE my job.*

Five-year-old Lewis came in with his 7-year-old sister, Cicely. Not sure how we got on this topic, but Cicely started describing the color of Lewis's hair. She said it is a 'dirty blond'. Lewis immediately said with tears in his eyes, "that's not a nice thing to say." He later calmed down and asked me, "Can I take you out to dinner."

*This request was a first for me, this is beyond Cougar. I gingerly declined his offer.*

Six-year-old Alexis came in to see me because her mother needed to know if she had allergies. She had the classic symptoms- running itchy nose, watery eyes, and constant sneezing when outdoors. When I examined her, I noticed she had 'allergic shiners', aka- dark circles under her eyes.

I showed Alexis's mother the dark circles. Alexis immediately said, "just like yours?"

*I just went home that evening and put on extra night cream on my eyes.*

If there was going to be a Mr. Jude, this next patient was a close 2nd
(Joke, not for a middle-aged woman).

Seven-year-old Braylen was coming in every month for some illness or lack of one. 1st a bike accident, with a scratched knee, then a thorn in his foot, cough, and this day he came in because he threw up once. I examined Braylen and told him he was totally healthy, not dehydrated and would be simply fine. I tried reverse psychology and told him I could not keep seeing him every month because I need him healthy. Braylen replied, "I'll throw myself in a bottomless pit if I cannot see you again."

*Can someone call 9-1-1? Braylen went on to stay very healthy. The visits became less frequent, like once every other month, and Braylen is alive.*

## Be as Innocent as a Child

Twelve-year-old Faith was being evaluated for possible Lyme disease. She had gotten bitten by a tick and was brave enough to remove it by herself. I asked Faith after she took the tick off her skin did it look irritated. She had a puzzled look on her face and then asked, "the tick?"

I take the blame, I failed to expand on what I was asking. I meant to ask Faith if her skin was irritated.

FYI- most people do not even know a tick has bitten them because it looks like a tiny mole on the skin. So, I instruct the parents to do head-to-toe surveillance every night at bath time by rubbing their hands on their child's skin. If they come across a raised bump, it probably is a tick, especially if it moves, and I am sure the tick is 'irritated', so get it off as soon as possible.

His father brought 11-year-old Jerry in because he had failing grades and probably had ADHD. The father explained to me that the school would not provide extra services for students without a documented diagnosis. I asked the father if Jerry did get a diagnosis of ADHD will he get an AID. Jerry yells out, "Great, first I have ADHD, now I have AIDS."

Five-year-old Henry- during his annual physical, going over developmental questions:
Can you count to 10? Answer: Yes, I can count to 99
Can you tie your shoelace? Answer: yes, I can
Can you ride a bike? Response: yes, with training wheels
Can you skip? Answer: Skip what?

Five-year-old Jackson came in for his Kindergarten physical. To assess his gross motor skills, I asked him if he knew how to skip. He said yes. So, I told him to skip. Jackson said, "1, 3, 5, 7."

Five-year-old Aurora came in for her Kindergarten physical, I asked her if she had a great summer, she said she did. So, I asked if she had gone to the beach, she again said yes. I asked if she had gone to Ocean City (one of the best beaches in Maryland). She said yes and stated, "I went to the ocean, and when I turned around the city was right there."

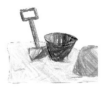

Four-year-old Angela told me about her birthday party and that she got a Barbie car. She stated that her friend Megan came to the party but was driving her new barbie car fast. I asked if Megan wrecked it. Angela corrected me and stated, 'no, no, she did not have a hammer."

*No more Mario games for Angela.*

A family of 3 (12, 9 and 6 years old) came in because the 9-year-old was experiencing ear pain. I diagnosed him with an ear infection and prescribed an antibiotic. I then instructed the Mother that the 9-year-old should not swim or fly for a few weeks due to fluid buildup in the middle ear canal. The Mother informed me that the family was going out of state for the grandmother's college graduation, but due to this recent diagnosis, she will have to stay home with the 9-year-old. The 6-year-old stated, "Dad is going, so the mother said, "yes, but do not tell Grandmother because she does not know; it is going to be a surprise." The 12-year-old shouts, "Grandma does not know she is graduating from college?"

**Culinary Preferences in Kids**

During 6 -year-old Xavier's physical examination, I asked about his food selections.
Do you like vegetables? Answer: "yes, carrots."
Do you like fruits? Answer: "yes, apples."
Do you like meats? Answer: "yes, not human meat, only animal meat, like pig."

*Good, because I did not like the movie, "Silence of the Lambs"*

Five-year-old Robert told me about his friend, Zion, a vegetarian. He said he does not like meat; he only eats vegetables, like corn dogs.

Five-year-old Drew. I asked what his favorite food is. He answered, "Can I say my favorite junk food? Coco Puffs."

Five-year-old Ashley came in for her physical and booster shots. She looked very terrified. Her Mother reassured her after shots she will get a dessert. Ashley answered. "This is a really tough decision, SHOTS or DESSERTS."

During 5-year-old Cain's physical exam, I notice his BMI (Body Mass Index) was slightly elevated, as was his weight percentile, so I asked Cain if he likes Fast food. He replied sheepishly; "well, I usually eat a little fast."

Four-year-old Ruth was asked what her favorite meat was. She replied: "My favorite chicken nugget is from Chick-fil-a, and my 2nd favorite is from a real chicken."

*Sorry Chick-fil-a, this is from the mouth of babes.*

I asked 7-year-old Jack what his favorite food is. He states it is Watermelon. He tells me he wrote a paper for school entitled "What is my favorite fruit to take on a field trip." He was so proud he stated it was 3 pages long. I could not imagine what a 7-year-old could write on watermelon for 3 pages. So, he summarized what he wrote: 1st- watermelon is 85% water, 2nd- it cost 68 cents at Walmart, 3rd-you do not have to throw anything away. You can just put the rind in your Tupperware and take back to school.

*Bravo, I would give him a A+++.*

6-year-old Don came in for his well visit. I asked about his dietary preferences.

What is your favorite food? Don's answer: Mac-n-cheese.

Favorite fruit. Answer: Apple.

Favorite meat. Answer: Chicken.

Favorite vegetable: Answer: NOTHING.

## Your Majesty

Four-year-old Vicky came in for a physical and did not want to get on the examination table to be examined. She adamantly objected. Her mother asked if she wanted her to hold her hand. She agreed. After getting on the table, she asked me; "can I have a pillow."

## My Fashion Critics

Being in medicine, I try and dress professionally and conservatively. On this day, I felt a bit adventurous and decided to wear a shoe with leopard spots on the top. 6-year-old Aiden walked into the room who immediately asked me if I was a wearing Cheetah girl shoe. After examining Aiden, his Mother brought his 4-year-old sister into the room for her examination, and he whispers to her, "Dr. Jude is wearing Cheetah girl shoes." I went home that day and trash those shoes.

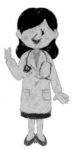

Nine-year-old Fred came in for his 1st visit. When I walked into the room, he states, "wow you're huge." His father welcomed me to give him a lot of shots because 'he called you huge,' he said. Just for clarification, I am 5ft 11 inches and wear a size 6 dress size. I would not be called huge by any stretched of the imagination. Tall but not huge.

*Thank you very much. I just needed to clarify that.*

I love my autistic patients because they are brutally honest. Thank God I have a great self-esteem. I guess Finn had not watch any Jackson Five videos from the 70s or the short film - 'Hair love' which won an Oscar in 2019.

I mention color, ethnicity, and hair types due to the punch line, so please keep reading. 7-year-old Finn is a Caucasian male who has autism. He came in to see me for referral renewals. I had not seen him in over a year. His mother had straight blond hair. As an African American I had been wearing my hair in a curly natural puff, which I love. Finn's mother asked him if he remembered me, as it had been over a year since our last encounter. Finn answered, with a scowl on his face "it is hard to forget her, with a hair like that."

*Love you Finn*

**Concept of Time**

Six-year-old Angie came in for a sick visit. I asked her if anything hurts. She responds, "I still had a headache for a couple of years now."

One of my favorite patients, 10-year-old Guy came in for a sick visit; he had a fever and cold. I checked out his birthday and told him he and my father have the same name and the same birthday, trying to make a close connection

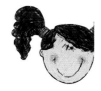

since he is one of my favorites. Guy answered, "maybe he was born on the same day as me or maybe a year before me."

## Concept of money

6-year-old Lia just lost her 1st two teeth and told me she received $2.00. She was so excited as she told me she was almost rich now.

## The wonder of imaginary play

Imaginary play is very crucial for the developing brain. I inform the patients and their parents that studies have shown that if kids are on electronics devices for more than 2 hours/ day, it decreases their ability to develop these critical abilities to reason and create, along with other higher cortical functions. I find fewer kids are using their brains to establish creativity which could serve them well in their academic studies and life.

There are always exceptions to the rule as seen with 4-year-old Jefferson.

I asked him if he plays make-believe. Jefferson said," yes I do, but nothing changes, nothing changes, nothing changes." And then he demonstrated, moving his hands in circles (like a magician). "See," he said, "nothing happened."

**Fiction vs Non-fiction**

Five-year-old Peter was about to travel to California on vacation. I asked if he was going to visit his Grandparents. He corrected me and stated that his grandmother does not live in California, just his Fairy Godmother.

**The Rewards of Parenting**

Seven-year-old Ruth came in for a physical. I went over safety questions, and the last question I asked was, "what would you do if you went to the store with your parents and suddenly you could not find them." Ruth's answer is, "be happy."

*I think Ruth had to walk home that day.*

I was doing a Kindergarten physical on 5-year-old Anthony, bringing along his 3-year-old sister and 7-year-old brother. I asked the same safety question regarding what he would do if he went to the store with his family and could not find them. As he pondered his answer, his 3-year-old sister, Desie, blasted out, "get a new family."

A 12-year-old Randy came in for his booster shots in preparation for the upcoming school year. I told him he needed 2 shots. Randy then totally lost it. He screamed his head off, causing such a stir in the clinic. After screaming and crying for a few minutes, his mother told Randy he was acting like a baby. He yelled back, "I AM a baby."

Randy can use advise from 13-year-old Watson, who told me his trick for not feeling pain when he gets vaccines; he recites the alphabet backwards, "It numbs the pain Doc."

**It is Stressful Being a Kindergartener**

Five-year-old Susan came in because she was often urinating, so her mother wanted to rule out a urinary tract infection. The laboratory test returned negative, and all other contributing factors were negative. I figured that Susan must be a bit stressed, so I asked her if she had been worried at home or school. She answered yes. Little Susan told me another kindergartener called her names on the school bus. I asked what he called her. She said he call me a "DUCK."

Five-and-a-half-year-old Maria came in for her Kindergarten physical. She looked a bit concerned, so I asked if anything bothered her about starting Kindergarten. She said, "yes, …. the big kids."

Five-year-old Chloe was telling me about kindergarten. I asked what her teacher's name was. She said, "her name is Ms. Hart, but she has no heart; she is not nice."

**Kids love to talk about intestinal and urination issues.**

Seven-year-old Maggie came in for a physical. I asked if she goes to the bathroom regularly for # 1 and #2. She said yes and even #3. I asked what #3 is. She said is starts with a "d … diarrhea."

Nine-year-old Kathleen came along with her newborn baby sister for her 1st doctor's visit. Kathleen was very proud to be a big sister. I asked if she prayed for a baby sister or baby brother when her mother was pregnant. Kathleen quickly informed me she was praying for a sister because a brother would have too many poopies.

Six-year-old Charles. I asked if he had any problems going to the potty. He replied, "ooh, sometimes I stand up."

During the general physical examination, I must examine all body parts. I try to tell the kids the different body parts I am about to examine. To respect a child's privacy, I reassure them I am a doctor, their mother or father is right there, and nothing terrible will happen. When examining the genitalia, I will use the appropriate terminology to explain what I am about to do (that is age appropriate).

I was about to examine 4-year-old Mark genitalia, so I told him, "I have to take a look at your underwear to ensure everything is there." Mark responds, "you don't have to look, my underwear is still there."

Twelve-year-old Ashley came for an evaluation of vaginal discharge. I explained to her I needed to get a culture of the discharge. She states, "it is not the prettiest site."

Seven-year-old Anton came in for a physical. I asked him if he had any problems going to the potty. He said yes. I asked what happened. Anton stated, "I stand up, peep on the toilet, then clean it up."

Another family with a 4-year-old son was asked the same question. Robert said he was not having any problems going to the potty. "I don't have to take any toys or my iPhone or iPad, I just poop."

Eleven-year-old Amelia just started her menstrual cycle. When asked how she was dealing with it, she said it feels like "Flaming hot Cheetos diarrhea".

*Sorry for the graphic nature. Kids truly are brutally honest.*

Five-year-old Lincoln came in for a physical. While I was asking developmental questions, he passed gas (flatus). His mother was so embarrassed she asked Lincoln, "what are you supposed to say." Lincoln said, "you're welcome."

Four-year-old Elijah was brought in by his mother who needed help with potty training. She stated she was so frustrated because Elijah feared the toilet, "he will not peep in it, he only peeps on trees."

I was doing a physical for a timid 6-year-old boy, accompanied by his mother and 9-year-old brother. I asked the 6-year-old about his bowel movement; "is it hard or soft." In the background, I heard the 9-year-old brother say," he can't touch it."

*Okay, enough poop, peep, underwear statements. I am sure there will be a few more.*

*Sorry, I just found a few more.*

Five-year-old Ian came in for his annual physical. I noted he was an adorable, polite young man. I asked him if he had any problems with # 1 or #2. He politely stated, "no, no problems with peep, poop or farts."

Three-year-old Elliot came in with his mother for his brother's well baby examination. While finishing up the baby's appointment, I notice Elliot was pulling at his pants, so I asked him if he needed to go to the potty. He said, 'no, I want to go to the tree."

Eight-year-old Ray came in for a routine physical. I asked about his diet; his mother told me he was a picky eater and does not like vegetables or fruits. I tried encouraging him to eat vegetables and fruits to avoid developing constipation. Ray asked me what constipation is. I told him it is when his poopies got hard, so I asked him if they were hard. Ray answered, "I don't know, because I don't feel them".

*Ok, one more.*

I promise, I kept the best for last. A bit of background information for the next patient encounter. A clinic or hospital has different emergency codes that are in place for the safety of everyone. Like a Code Red is for Fire, Code Blue is Cardiac/Respiratory arrest, Code Black is Bomb threat, etc. The following Code is very critical in Pediatrics. Code Pink is for Infant or Child Abduction. If a Code Pink is called, the entire clinic/hospital shuts down until the child/infant is found.

I almost activated Code Pink during this next family visit.

A family of 3 kids; 14, 11 and 9 years old, all came in for refills on ADHD medications. The 9-year-old decided he needed to go to the bathroom right after I walked into the exam room, so I directed him to the bathroom down the hallway as I returned to exam his siblings. He was gone for a while, so I send the 11-year-old to find out where he was. The 11-year-old also did not come back promptly. I was a bit nervous, so I left the exam room to find these two possible missing kids. I find the 11-year-old leisurely watching TV in the Waiting Room while the 9-year-old remained in the bathroom. The 9-year-old eventually came out of the bathroom and rejoin his family in the exam room. I ask him if he got sick, he said no. I asked if he had diarrhea or threw up. He said no. I told the family I was very concerned and almost activated a Code pink. I asked the 9-year-old if he knew what Code Pink was? The 11-year sister immediately answers, "DIARRHEA."

**Parents should be so proud of their little ones.**

Four-year-old Jimmy came in for his wellness visit. I wanted to assess his developmental milestones, so I asked him if he could sing a song. He said no. I said, can you sing ABCs? He said, "no." Twinkle, twinkle little stars? He again said "no." Mary had a little lamb. "No again," Jimmy said. He said I could sing, "Bubba, Bubba, don't shoot the jukebox, O Bubba, Bubba, please don't shoot the jukebox."

*There He is - The Next Willie Nelson.*

Eight-year-old Ali came in to see me complaining of right ear pain. I diagnosed him with Swimmer's ear and prescribed ear drops. I informed the mother the drops should not burn or sting but if it did to put in the refrigerator. Ali eyes grew huge, and he said, "please don't put me in the refrigerator."

I asked 4-year-old Anna about doing chores during her well visit. I asked if she cleans up her room and pick up her toys. She replies, "Yes, only if people are coming over."

**The Next Sigmond Freud**

Three-year-old Nathan, I was trying to assess his ability to understand deductive reasoning and contrast during his physical exam, so I asked him, "are you hot or cold". His answer was "warm."

**Watch out world, your job is secure with our up-and-coming professionals.**

Eight-year-old Katie came in for her annual physical exam. I asked her what she wanted to do when she got older. Her answered: 1ˢᵗ a doctor, 2ⁿᵈ a Vegetarian.

*Watch out animals. Katie might be fixing all your illnesses and aches with vegetables. She meant to say Veterinarian.*

**To die or not to dye**

Josh came in for his PreK physical along with his two older brothers. 11 and 9-year-old brothers, Sam, and Chris. Sam and Josh's hair color was brunette, and middle brother, Chris was blonde like his mother. The mother went on to state how interesting genetics is because the middle son, Chris, took after her family, all blondes, while Sam and Josh took after the father's family. I was curious as I noticed the mother's hair was also brunette. She read my mind and stated that she was a blonde during childhood but dyed her hair while in college. Josh went over and hugged his mom tightly as he said, "I didn't know you died."

**Kid love chores-right.**

Doing chores is an important part of childhood as it teaches the child responsibility, helps improve fine and gross motor skills, helps teach respect for their parents, and the ability to follow rules, along with many other great attributes. 7-year-old Sierra was asked during her physical if she does chores at home, and she answered no. She had told me earlier that she has a cat who sleeps with her. I asked Sierra if she could feed her cat. She said No. So, I asked if she gave her cat water. Before she could answer, I said "I

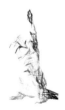

know, no, the cat probably gets her water". Sierra raised her arms while on the exam table and demonstrated saying emphatically "CATS DO NOT HAVE HANDS".

*I guess she told me.*

The Jetson was a futuristic cartoon series from the 60s and 70s that featured flying cars, Robotics that talked and cleaned the house, also a vacuum that cleaned the carpet.

Today in clinic in the 21st century, 2021, I did a Kindergarten physical for a set of adorable twins, Oli, and Wyatt. I asked Wyatt if he had a dog or a cat, he answered, "No, just a vacuum cleaner."

Seven-year-old Patty answers to the anticipatory guidelines during her annual visit.
What grade are you in? Answer: 2nd grade
What was your favorite subject in 1st grade? Answer: Nothing
What do you want to do when you become an adult? Answer: Stay at home.

**The love for school**

During 9-year-old Ryan's physical examination, I asked if he had any problems falling asleep. Mom's answer: No, when the lights go out, he is out. Ryan immediately states, 'but not at school". I went on to ask if he brushes his teeth once or twice. His answer: "both."

*(Smart aleck)*

Eight-year-old Mickey came in to get an evaluation for ADHD. His mother stated Mickey is a brilliant student and gets all As and Bs, but gets "I" for homework. I asked what "I" signifies. The mother stated," incomplete." Mickey replied, "No, it means impossible."

Seven-year-old Calvin came in for a physical exam the Monday after school was over for the year. He had just completed 1$^{st}$ grade and had passed to the 2$^{nd}$ grade, so I asked him what he enjoyed about 1$^{st}$ grade. Answer: "the last day."

I hope this next patient will not be one of those waitresses at Hooters

Eight-year-old Summer came in for her annual physical. She was laying on her back while I palpated her chest to assess if she had started puberty. We use the Tanner staging to evaluate stages of puberty. I informed the mother that there were no signs of puberty, and her Tanner stage was at 1, meaning no breast development. The patient quickly asked if I could check her breast while she laid on her side.

*Sorry Summer, front, back or side, there are NO breast, nada, zero.*

## The Honest of Kids

Ten-year-old Martha came in with Upper respiratory symptoms: cough, nasal congestion, decrease appetite, and energy level. I explained to the mother the treatment is supportive as I explained to her the details. The mother stated she was already doing those measures by keeping Martha hydrated with lots of fluids and just keeping her in bed. Martha responded, "but I have been on the couch."

Six-year-old Heather just had her eye test done (the Snellen test). I informed her that she failed the test and might need eyeglasses. Heather said: "yes because I had to cover one eye, but I use to using two eyes to see."

Fourteen-year-old Pippa was having problems concentrating in school, so I referred her to a psychologist. After a few sessions, she came back to see me for something else. I asked her how the therapy was going. She said, "terribly because all the therapist does is talk about herself and does not allow me to state my concerns." Pippa now knows that her therapist has Multiple sclerosis and learns about her victories in sport and family drama. Pippa then states she does not need to go back because she gets all that drama during lunch at Middle school, but at least she gets a sandwich and salad.

Fourteen-year-old Chrislene started working on the weekends by babysitting and walking the dogs in her neighborhood. She proudly told me she quit the baby-sitting job and kept the dog walking business because she got paid more for the dogs than the humans.

Jack came in for his annual physical exam. I remembered him because I had just seen him three weeks earlier and he was only four years old. Jack was talking up a storm during this visit; he was very articulate and not at all shy. I could not believe how mature he had gotten in such a short time. I told him I could not believe he was now five years old, because just the other day, he was 4. I asked him, "when did you turn 5". He answered, "on my birthday."

Six-year-old Mark came in to be evaluated for fever and diarrhea episodes, rapidly resolving. He smiled throughout the visit and seemed to return to his usual happy self. He became very excited after I examined him and told him he was better. He chimes in and tells me, "I got a $100 bill from my Great Grandfather for my birthday and then he DIED!!!

*Okayyy??*

Nine-year-old Axel came in for anger issues because his parents were going through a divorce. I had to ensure he was stable and not a threat to himself or others, so I asked him a few questions. I asked him if he felt suicidal. He asked what that meant. Being he was only nine years old and naïve, I did not want to sound so morbid, so I rephrase the question and asked, "do you feel like hurting yourself." Axel replied, "yes, I'll do it right now." He then punched himself in the face.

*I was so stunt I couldn't say a word. After getting over the shock of seeing this WWF move, I immediately referred him to Behavioral Health ASAP.*

Five-year-old Juan come in for his kindergarten physical. He was very academically advanced. Juan could count to 1000 and write his 1st and last name and his brother's name. I complimented him on how smart he was and told him he needed to be in 1st grade. He said, "o no, I'm staying in Kindergarten to have more fun". I went on to ask him a safety question if he knew how to ride a bike. Juan said, "yes, but I just never tried."

**Watch Out for Mr. Don Juan**

Twelve-year-old Fred came in because he told his parents one of his testicles was larger than the other. To provide privacy, I closed the shades on the windows; as the father said: "I don't think the birds give a hoot." After laughing for a few minutes, I examined Fred and discovered that one of his testicles was larger than the other, probably due to the onset of uberty.

While typing up his note, I realized it was his birthday, so I asked him why he came in on his birthday to have this type of exam (I thought it would be embarrassing and humiliating). Fred yelled out, "This was the best birthday ever."

### Children have the World Figured Out

Concerned about sibling rivalry, I asked 12-year-old Margaret if she gets along with her 10-year-old sister because they had been arguing throughout the entire visit. I explained to her that she needs to be nice to her sister because they will be together longer than their parents. Ms. Margaret politely told me: "I get along with my sister, we already plan to live together after our kids have moved out and our husbands are dead."

*I did not know if I should run out the room and call my only sister, who is older than me and who I have looked up to all my life and tell her, "Change of plans."*

Nine-year-old Marcus came in for his annual examination. His mother was very concerned and wanted her son tested for dyslexia. She stated she wants Marcus to learn coping skills to deal with this possible disability. Marcus replies, "is it like a shock collar for dogs?"

### Kids Really do get Sick

One of the many reasons I love kids is they are so resilient, even when sick. It can get confusing and challenging because they may have a fever but still run around in the clinic. So, when 10-year-old Rachel came in with flu-like symptoms, cough, sore throat, and fever, she looked so uncomfortable, I asked her how she felt. "I feel like dog poop," she said. Her response brought tears to my eyes.

Thirteen-year-old Lynsee came in due to an episode of sneezing, cough, and watery eyes for a few months. She had a history of Allergic rhinitis and was treated with Zyrtec (an allergy medication). Mom felt the drug was not working. I informed the mother I would prescribe another allergy medication to control her symptoms better. Still, if this medication did not work, I would need to consider giving her allergy shots. Lynsee asked, "what is that." I told her, "You don't want to know." She turned to her mother and tears and asked, "Am I going to die?"

Five-year-old Tommy came in with a croupy cough. The medical description of this type of cough is a barking cough. I asked Tommy why he came in today. He replied, "I have a dog cough."

**The effects of the COVID Pandemic**

Seven-year-old Bertha came in for her annual physical exam. She passed her vision scream and scored well 20/20. I told Bertha she did a great job. She looked relieved and told me she thought she did 'bad' because 2020 was a bad year.

**Last entry** but not the last encounter in my career. This was the icing on the cake that solidified my decision to pursue pediatrics.

His father brought 5-year-old Dylan in for a physical. I showed him where his heart was located on his chest because he was very curious about his body; right under his left breast, and told him what the heart sounds like-"lub dub, lub dub." Dylan asked me with a cute smile, "do you want to know what my heart sounds like, Dr. Jude?" I answered 'sure." Dylan answered, it says "I love you; I love you."

I hope you laughed as much as I did and can appreciate the beauty of childhood filled with innocence, wonder and laughter. I hope the parents also gleaned a few pointers on child's health and treatment options, as those medical pearls were hidden in plain sight throughout the book.

I love teaching parents how to care for their little and older ones, even if used through comedy. **Proverbs 17: 22** sums it up best: A cheerful heart is good medicine.

A famous person who I have loved and admired all my life once stated,

*"If you enter this world knowing that you are loved and leave this world knowing the same, then everything that happens in between can be dealt with"*

Michael Jackson

*Miss you my love, your 'Liberian girl'*

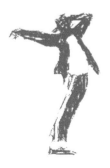

# ACKNOWLEDGEMENT

I thank my patients for providing me the raw materials for this book, without which this book would not have been possible (literally). Most of the names were altered, but if you were one of my patients and one of these famous quotes is yours, please know that you are indeed a star, designed for greatness, beyond your imagination.

A hearty thanks to my sister, Bijou Jude Butler for the beautiful picture she created for this book's cover after I just gave her an idea of what I wanted.

I don't think there will be a second book on this topic because I will NOT be working another 25 years to collect materials.

Thank you very much.

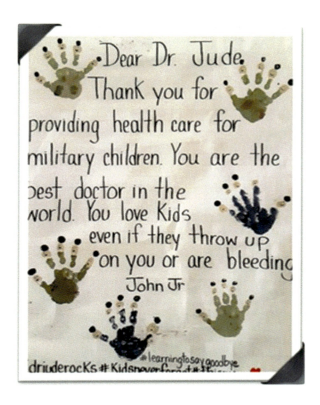

Dear Dr. Jude, Thank you for providing health care for military children. You are the best doctor in the world. You love kids even if they throw up on you or are bleeding. John Jr

drjuderocks #Kidsnever... #learningtosaygoodbye

At that time the disciples came to Jesus and asked, "Who, then, is the greatest in the kingdom of heaven?" He called a little child to him, and placed the child among them, And He said: "Truly I tell you, unless you change and become like little children, you will never enter the kingdom of heaven. Therefore, whoever takes the lowly position of this child is greatest in the kingdom of heaven. And whoever welcomes one such child in my name welcomes me.

Matthew 18: 1-5

## ABOUT THE AUTHOR

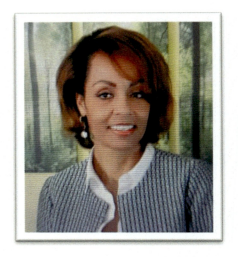

Dr. Bonita L. Jude is a Board-Certified Pediatrician, who lives in Silver Spring, Maryland and works in military medicine with the Department of Health Agency. Dr. Jude is also the author of PURITY, a handbook designed to teach girls and young ladies to live a life of Purity for God's kingdom, for their fulfillment and protection.

Dr. Jude is available to teach the PURITY course to schools, church groups and is available to speak at Parents conferences/ seminars. Her desire is for the younger generation to live out their God given desires and destinies, despite obstacles, challenges, or detours.

Though not initially clear, Bonita shouts for joy that the Lord allowed her life to be an Isaish 54 woman.

Contact information: Pedshousecall@gmail.com

*You did it again Abba Father.*
*Another dream accomplished to give you glory and honor.*

Printed in the United States
by Baker & Taylor Publisher Services